POLYMYALGIA RHEUMATICA DIET

Nourish Your Body, Relieve Pain and Improve Mobility

Sharon D. Hayden

CONTENTS

PREFACE

Welcome to "Polymyalgia Rheumatica Diet"!

Polymyalgia rheumatica (PMR) is a chronic inflammatory condition that causes pain, stiffness, and discomfort, primarily in the shoulders, hips, and neck. Managing the symptoms of PMR can be challenging, but adopting a well-planned and balanced diet can play a crucial role in alleviating inflammation, reducing pain, and improving overall well-being.

This book serves as a comprehensive guide to understanding the Polymyalgia Rheumatica Diet. Whether you have recently been diagnosed with PMR or have been living with the condition for some time, this book will provide you with the knowledge, strategies, and practical tips to optimize your diet and enhance your quality of life.

Throughout the pages of this book, you will discover the importance of nutrition in managing PMR and promoting overall health. From understanding the inflammatory nature of certain foods to identifying nutrient-rich options, from incorporating anti-inflammatory ingredients into your meals to managing potential dietary triggers, each chapter is designed to equip you with the tools and insights you need to make informed decisions about your diet.

I have compiled this book based on scientific research, expert opinions, and my own experiences. However, it is essential to remember that each person's body and health circumstances are unique. What works for one individual may not be suitable for another. Therefore, I encourage you to listen to your body, tailor the dietary recommendations to fit your specific needs, and seek personalized guidance from healthcare professionals.

As you embark on your journey with the Polymyalgia Rheumatica Diet, I encourage you to approach it with an open mind and a commitment to your well-being. Remember that the journey to managing PMR involves more than just dietary modifications; it is a holistic approach that encompasses various aspects of self-care, including exercise, stress management, and medication adherence.

I hope that this book will serve as a valuable resource, guiding you towards a healthier and more fulfilling life despite the challenges of PMR. May it empower you to make informed choices about your diet, inspire you to embrace a proactive approach to your health, and ultimately contribute to your overall well-being.

Best wishes,

INTRODUCTION

Polymyalgia rheumatica (PMR) is a chronic inflammatory disorder that primarily affects individuals over the age of 50. It is characterized by pain, stiffness, and inflammation in the muscles, particularly around the shoulders, neck, hips, and thighs. PMR is often accompanied by general malaise, fatigue, and a low-grade fever. The exact cause of PMR is unknown, but it is believed to involve an autoimmune response, where the body's immune system mistakenly attacks its own tissues.

PMR is more common in women than men and typically occurs in individuals of Northern European descent. The condition tends to develop gradually, with symptoms worsening over time. The pain and stiffness experienced in PMR can be debilitating and severely impact an individual's quality of life.

The diagnosis of PMR is primarily based on clinical evaluation and exclusion of other possible causes of musculoskeletal symptoms. Medical history, physical examination, and laboratory tests play a crucial role in the diagnosis. Blood tests may reveal elevated levels of markers of inflammation, such as erythrocyte sedimentation rate (ESR) and C-reactive protein (CRP). Imaging tests, such as ultrasound or magnetic resonance imaging (MRI), may be used to assess the extent of inflammation in the affected muscles and rule out other conditions.

Treatment for PMR usually involves the use of corticosteroids, such as prednisone, which help reduce inflammation and alleviate symptoms. The initial dosage of corticosteroids is often high and gradually tapered down over time. Regular monitoring is essential to adjust the dosage and minimize potential side effects associated with long-term corticosteroid use. In some cases, other immunosuppressive medications may be prescribed to reduce the reliance on corticosteroids.

Overall, PMR is a chronic condition that requires long-term management to control symptoms and maintain quality of life. While there is no known cure for PMR, proper medical care and lifestyle adjustments can help individuals with PMR lead fulfilling lives.

Symptoms And Diagnosis Of Pmr

PMR is characterized by several key symptoms that

primarily affect the musculoskeletal system. The most common symptoms include:

1. **Pain and Stiffness**: Individuals with PMR often experience moderate to severe pain and stiffness, particularly in the shoulders, neck, hips, and thighs. These symptoms are typically more pronounced in the morning or after periods of inactivity.

2. **Limited Range of Motion**: The stiffness associated with PMR can lead to a limited range of motion in the affected joints. Simple tasks like lifting the arms or getting out of bed may become challenging.

3. **General Malaise and Fatigue**: Many individuals with PMR experience a sense of general malaise and fatigue. This can be attributed to the underlying inflammation and the body's immune response.

4. **Low-Grade Fever**: Some individuals with PMR may have a low-grade fever, typically below 100.4°F (38°C).

Diagnosing PMR requires a comprehensive evaluation of symptoms, medical history, and laboratory tests. Since the symptoms of PMR can overlap with other conditions, it is crucial to rule out alternative causes of musculoskeletal pain and stiffness. The diagnosis process often includes:

1. **Medical History**: The doctor will inquire about the nature, duration, and severity of symptoms. They will also consider the patient's medical history, including any previous autoimmune or

rheumatic diseases.

2. **Physical Examination**: The doctor will perform a physical examination to assess the range of motion in the affected joints and muscles. They may also look for signs of inflammation, such as redness or swelling.

3. **Blood Tests**: Laboratory tests, including ESR and CRP, are commonly used to measure the levels of inflammation in the body. Additionally, blood tests may include the measurement of other markers, such as rheumatoid factor and anti-cyclic citrullinated peptide antibodies, to help rule out other inflammatory conditions like rheumatoid arthritis.

4. **Imaging Tests**: Imaging tests like ultrasound or MRI may be conducted to visualize the affected joints and muscles. These tests can help confirm the presence of inflammation and rule out other potential causes of symptoms.

5. **Response to Treatment**: One of the key factors in diagnosing PMR is the response to treatment with corticosteroids. If the symptoms improve significantly after starting corticosteroid therapy, it can be an indication of PMR.

It is important to note that there is no definitive diagnostic test for PMR, and the diagnosis is based on a combination of clinical evaluation, exclusion of other conditions, and response to treatment. A rheumatologist, a specialist in musculoskeletal and autoimmune disorders, is often involved in the diagnosis and management of PMR.

Early and accurate diagnosis of PMR is crucial to initiate appropriate treatment and minimize the impact of the condition on daily life.

Impact Of Diet On Pmr Management

While there is no specific diet that has been proven to cure or directly treat PMR, adopting a healthy and balanced diet can play a supportive role in managing the condition and overall well-being. Here are some key considerations regarding diet and PMR management:

1. **Anti-inflammatory Foods**: Including anti-inflammatory foods in the diet may help reduce overall inflammation in the body. These foods include fruits and vegetables (especially berries, leafy greens, and cruciferous vegetables), fatty fish rich in omega-3 fatty acids (such as salmon and mackerel), nuts and seeds, and healthy fats from sources like olive oil and avocados.

2. **Low-Processed, Whole Foods**: A diet consisting of minimally processed, whole foods can provide essential nutrients, promote overall health, and support the immune system. It is advisable to limit the consumption of processed and refined foods, including sugary snacks, processed meats, and foods high in saturated and trans fats.

3. **Adequate Protein Intake**: Protein is essential for muscle health and repair. Including lean sources of protein, such as poultry, fish, legumes,

and tofu, can help support muscle function in individuals with PMR. It is important to consult with a healthcare professional or registered dietitian to determine the appropriate protein intake for individual needs.

4. **Maintaining a Healthy Weight**: Excess weight can place additional strain on joints and muscles, exacerbating the symptoms of PMR. Therefore, maintaining a healthy weight through a balanced diet and regular physical activity can help reduce the burden on the musculoskeletal system.

5. **Individualized Approach**: It is important to recognize that the impact of diet on PMR management can vary from person to person. Some individuals may find certain foods trigger or worsen their symptoms, while others may not experience significant changes. Keeping a food diary and monitoring individual responses can help identify any personal dietary triggers or patterns.

While diet can be a complementary component of PMR management, it should not replace medical treatment or prescribed medications. It is essential to work with healthcare professionals, such as rheumatologists and dietitians, to develop a comprehensive management plan that addresses individual needs and goals.

CHAPTER ONE

Understanding the Role

of Diet in PMR

Polymyalgia rheumatica (PMR) is an inflammatory condition that primarily affects older adults. It is characterized by stiffness and pain in the muscles, particularly in the shoulders, neck, and hips. While the exact cause of PMR is unknown, research suggests that diet plays a significant role in managing the symptoms and reducing inflammation. A well-balanced, anti-inflammatory diet can help alleviate pain, improve overall health, and enhance the effectiveness of medical treatments. This article explores the relationship between diet and PMR, highlighting the inflammatory nature of the condition and the importance of adopting an anti-inflammatory diet for managing PMR effectively.

Inflammatory Nature Of Pmr

PMR is classified as an autoimmune disorder, which means

that the body's immune system mistakenly attacks its own tissues. In the case of PMR, the immune system targets the synovial membranes, which are responsible for lubricating the joints. This immune response leads to inflammation in the affected areas, resulting in pain and stiffness. The underlying mechanism behind PMR's inflammatory nature involves the release of pro-inflammatory cytokines, such as tumor necrosis factor-alpha (TNF-α) and interleukin-6 (IL-6). These cytokines promote inflammation and contribute to the characteristic symptoms experienced by individuals with PMR.

Connection Between Diet And Inflammation

Research has shown that diet can have a profound impact on the body's inflammatory response. Certain foods can either promote or reduce inflammation, making dietary choices crucial for individuals with PMR. A diet high in processed foods, refined sugars, and unhealthy fats can contribute to chronic inflammation and exacerbate PMR symptoms. On the other hand, a diet rich in anti-inflammatory foods can help reduce inflammation, relieve pain, and improve overall well-being. By understanding the connection between diet and inflammation, individuals with PMR can make informed choices to better manage their condition.

Importance Of An Anti-Inflammatory Diet For Pmr

Adopting an anti-inflammatory diet is a key component of managing PMR effectively. Such a diet focuses on consuming foods that have been shown to have anti-inflammatory properties, while avoiding those that promote inflammation. Here are some essential points to consider when following an anti-inflammatory diet for PMR:

1. Increase Intake of Fruits and Vegetables: Fruits and vegetables are rich in antioxidants, vitamins, minerals, and fiber, all of which contribute to reducing inflammation. Aim to include a variety of colorful fruits and vegetables in your diet, such as berries, leafy greens, cruciferous vegetables, and citrus fruits.

2. Emphasize Omega-3 Fatty Acids: Omega-3 fatty acids, found in fatty fish (like salmon, sardines, and mackerel), flaxseeds, chia seeds, and walnuts, have powerful anti-inflammatory properties. Including these foods in your diet can help decrease inflammation and improve joint health.

3. Choose Whole Grains: Whole grains, such as quinoa, brown rice, oats, and whole wheat bread, contain fiber and other nutrients that help regulate inflammation in the body. Avoid refined grains, as they can spike blood sugar levels and promote inflammation.

4. Incorporate Healthy Fats: Healthy fats, such as those found in avocados, olive oil, nuts, and seeds, possess anti-inflammatory properties. These fats help reduce inflammation and provide essential nutrients for overall health. However, moderation is key, as they are high in calories.

5. Limit Processed Foods and Added Sugars: Processed foods, including fast food, packaged snacks, and sugary beverages, often contain unhealthy fats, added sugars, and artificial additives. These can trigger inflammation and worsen PMR symptoms. Opt for whole, unprocessed foods whenever possible, and reduce your intake of added sugars by avoiding sugary drinks and opting for natural sweeteners like honey or maple syrup instead.

6. Include Lean Protein Sources: Protein is an essential nutrient for tissue repair and immune function. Choose lean sources of protein such as skinless poultry, fish, legumes, and tofu. These options provide important amino acids without the added unhealthy fats found in processed meats.

7. Spice Up Your Meals: Certain spices and herbs have potent anti-inflammatory properties. Turmeric, ginger, garlic, and cinnamon, for example, have been shown to reduce inflammation in the body. Incorporate these spices into your meals to enhance flavor and provide potential anti-inflammatory benefits.

8. Stay Hydrated: Proper hydration is essential for overall health and can also help reduce inflammation. Drink an adequate amount of water throughout the day to support joint lubrication, digestion, and overall well-being.

9. Consider Food Sensitivities: Some individuals with PMR may have specific food sensitivities that can trigger inflammation and worsen symptoms. It can be helpful to work with a healthcare professional to identify any potential food sensitivities through an elimination diet or specific testing.

CHAPTER TWO

Polymyalgia rheumatica (PMR) is an inflammatory disorder characterized by muscle pain and stiffness, primarily affecting the shoulders, neck, and hips. While the exact cause of PMR is unknown, research suggests that certain nutrients can play a crucial role in managing its symptoms. One such group of nutrients is omega-3 fatty acids, which have been studied extensively for their potential benefits in various inflammatory conditions, including PMR. In this article, we will explore the sources of omega-3 fatty acids, their benefits for PMR, and the recommended intake and supplementation.

Omega-3 Fatty Acids:

Omega-3 fatty acids are a type of polyunsaturated fat that is essential for overall health. They are classified into three main types: alpha-linolenic acid (ALA), eicosapentaenoic acid (EPA), and docosahexaenoic acid (DHA). These fatty acids are not naturally produced by the body, so it is important to obtain them from dietary sources.

Sources Of Omega-3 Fatty Acids:

1. **Fatty Fish:** Fatty fish such as salmon, mackerel, sardines, and trout are excellent sources of EPA and DHA. These types of fish are considered the best dietary sources of omega-3 fatty acids.

2. **Flaxseeds and Chia Seeds:** Flaxseeds and chia seeds are plant-based sources of omega-3 fatty acids. They are rich in ALA, which can be converted into EPA and DHA in the body, although the conversion rate is limited.

3. **Walnuts:** Walnuts are a good source of ALA and also provide other beneficial nutrients such as fiber and antioxidants.

4. **Soybeans and Tofu:** Soybeans and tofu are plant-based sources of omega-3 fatty acids. They can be a great option for individuals who follow a vegetarian or vegan diet.

5. **Algal Oil:** Algal oil is derived from algae and is an excellent source of DHA. It is a suitable alternative for those who prefer not to consume fish or fish oil.

Benefits Of Omega-3 Fatty Acids For Pmr:

Omega-3 fatty acids have been studied for their potential anti-inflammatory effects, making them beneficial for managing PMR symptoms. Here are some of the potential benefits:

1. **Reduced Inflammation:** Omega-3 fatty acids can help reduce inflammation in the body by inhibiting the production of inflammatory substances called prostaglandins and leukotrienes. This anti-inflammatory effect may help alleviate the pain and stiffness associated with PMR.

2. **Joint Health:** PMR primarily affects the joints, causing pain and limited mobility. Omega-3 fatty acids may help support joint health by reducing inflammation and promoting the production of compounds that support joint structure and function.

3. **Cardiovascular Health:** PMR has been associated with an increased risk of cardiovascular diseases. Omega-3 fatty acids have been shown to have cardiovascular benefits, including reducing triglyceride levels, improving blood vessel function, and lowering blood pressure.

4. **Brain Health:** Omega-3 fatty acids, particularly DHA, are essential for brain health and development. They have been linked to improved

cognitive function and a reduced risk of neurodegenerative diseases. This is especially important for individuals with PMR, as they may be at a higher risk of cognitive impairment.

Recommended Intake And Supplementation:

The recommended intake of omega-3 fatty acids varies depending on age, sex, and health status. The American Heart Association (AHA) suggests the following guidelines:

- For healthy adults, consume at least two servings of fatty fish per week, with each serving providing about 250-500 milligrams (mg) of EPA and DHA combined.

- For individuals with PMR or other inflammatory conditions, higher doses of omega-3 fatty acids may be beneficial. Consult with a healthcare professional to determine the appropriate dosage.

Supplementation with omega-3 fatty acids is also an option for individuals who have difficulty obtaining enough through diet alone. Omega-3 supplements are available in the form of fish oil capsules, algal oil capsules (for vegetarian/vegan options), and flaxseed oil capsules. When choosing a supplement, it is important to look for products that have been third-party tested for purity and quality.

It is worth noting that omega-3 supplements should be used under the guidance of a healthcare professional, especially if you are taking any medications or have underlying health conditions. They can help determine the right dosage and ensure it is safe for you.

In addition to omega-3 fatty acids, it is important to maintain a balanced and nutritious diet to support overall health and manage PMR symptoms. Here are some additional dietary recommendations for individuals with PMR:

1. **Anti-Inflammatory Foods:** Include foods that have natural anti-inflammatory properties in your diet. These include fruits and vegetables, whole grains, nuts, seeds, and healthy fats like olive oil and avocados.

2. **Lean Protein:** Opt for lean sources of protein such as poultry, fish, legumes, and tofu. Protein is essential for muscle repair and maintenance.

3. **Calcium and Vitamin D:** PMR and its treatment can increase the risk of osteoporosis. Ensure an adequate intake of calcium and vitamin D to support bone health. Dairy products, fortified plant-based milks, leafy greens, and sunlight exposure are good sources of these nutrients.

4. **Hydration:** Stay hydrated by drinking plenty of water throughout the day. Proper hydration is important for joint and muscle health.

5. **Avoid Trigger Foods:** Some individuals with PMR may find that certain foods worsen their symptoms. Keep a food diary to identify any potential trigger foods, and work with a healthcare professional or registered dietitian to develop a personalized diet plan.

It is important to remember that dietary changes and supplements should not replace medical treatment for PMR. Always consult with a healthcare professional for a comprehensive treatment plan that addresses your specific needs

Antioxidants

Antioxidants are compounds that play a crucial role in maintaining the balance of free radicals in the body. Free radicals are highly reactive molecules that can cause oxidative stress, which is linked to various health issues, including chronic inflammation, aging, and certain diseases. Antioxidants help neutralize these free radicals, thus protecting the body's cells from damage. They are found in a wide range of foods and are also available as dietary supplements. Let's delve deeper into the types of antioxidants, foods rich in antioxidants, and the role of antioxidants in reducing inflammation.

Types Of Antioxidants

There are several types of antioxidants, each with its unique mechanism of action and sources. Here are some prominent types of antioxidants:

1. **Vitamin C (Ascorbic Acid):** Found abundantly

in fruits and vegetables, vitamin C is a powerful antioxidant that helps protect cells from oxidative damage. It also aids in the regeneration of other antioxidants in the body, such as vitamin E.

2. **Vitamin E (Tocopherol):** This fat-soluble vitamin is found in nuts, seeds, vegetable oils, and leafy greens. Vitamin E protects cell membranes from oxidative stress and works synergistically with vitamin C to enhance its antioxidant effects.

3. **Beta-carotene:** It is a precursor to vitamin A and acts as a potent antioxidant. Beta-carotene is commonly found in orange and yellow fruits and vegetables like carrots, sweet potatoes, and apricots.

4. **Selenium:** This essential mineral acts as a cofactor for certain antioxidant enzymes in the body. It is present in foods like Brazil nuts, seafood, whole grains, and eggs.

5. **Flavonoids:** Flavonoids are a diverse group of antioxidants found in many plant-based foods. Examples include quercetin (found in apples, onions, and berries) and catechins (found in green tea).

6. **Lycopene:** It is a carotenoid pigment that gives fruits like tomatoes and watermelons their red color. Lycopene exhibits potent antioxidant properties and is beneficial for cardiovascular health.

7. **Resveratrol:** Found in grapes, red wine, and berries, resveratrol is known for its antioxidant

and anti-inflammatory effects. It has gained attention for its potential role in promoting heart health.

Foods Rich In Antioxidants

Consuming a diverse range of antioxidant-rich foods is essential to ensure an adequate intake of these beneficial compounds. Here are some examples of foods that are particularly rich in antioxidants:

1. **Berries:** Blueberries, strawberries, raspberries, and blackberries are packed with various antioxidants, including vitamin C, flavonoids, and anthocyanins.

2. **Leafy Greens:** Spinach, kale, and Swiss chard are excellent sources of antioxidants, including vitamin C, vitamin E, and beta-carotene.

3. **Colorful Vegetables:** Bell peppers, tomatoes, carrots, and sweet potatoes are rich in antioxidants like vitamin C, beta-carotene, and lycopene.

4. **Nuts and Seeds:** Almonds, walnuts, flaxseeds, and chia seeds contain antioxidants such as vitamin E, selenium, and flavonoids.

5. **Green Tea:** Known for its high concentration of catechins, green tea is a popular antioxidant-rich beverage.

6. **Dark Chocolate:** Cocoa beans used to make dark chocolate are rich in flavonoids, including

procyanidins and epicatechins.

7. **Spices:** Turmeric, cinnamon, ginger, and cloves are spices known for their antioxidant properties.

It's important to note that a balanced diet consisting of a variety of whole foods is the best approach to ensure that you obtain a wide range of antioxidants from different sources. Incorporating these antioxidant-rich foods into your daily meals can contribute to maintaining optimal health and protecting against oxidative stress.

Role Of Antioxidants In Reducing Inflammation

Inflammation is a natural response of the body to injury or infection. However, when inflammation becomes chronic and persistent, it can contribute to the development of various diseases, including heart disease, diabetes, and certain types of cancer. Antioxidants play a significant role in reducing inflammation and mitigating its detrimental effects. Here's how antioxidants help in this regard:

1. **Neutralizing Free Radicals:** Free radicals can promote inflammation by damaging cells and triggering inflammatory responses. Antioxidants neutralize these free radicals, preventing them from causing further damage and reducing the inflammatory cascade.

2. **Inhibiting Pro-inflammatory Pathways:**

Antioxidants can interfere with the activation of pro-inflammatory molecules and pathways in the body. They can help modulate the production of inflammatory cytokines, enzymes, and signaling molecules, thereby reducing inflammation.

3. **Supporting the Immune System:** Antioxidants have been shown to support a healthy immune system, which plays a vital role in regulating inflammation. By maintaining immune balance, antioxidants can help prevent excessive and chronic inflammation.

4. **Protecting against Oxidative Stress:** Chronic inflammation is often accompanied by oxidative stress. Antioxidants counteract oxidative stress by neutralizing free radicals and preventing cellular damage. This protection against oxidative stress helps reduce inflammation and its associated complications.

5. **Enhancing Endogenous Antioxidant Systems:** Antioxidants not only act directly but also support the body's own antioxidant defense systems. For example, they can regenerate other antioxidants like vitamin E and glutathione, enhancing the overall antioxidant capacity of the body.

6. **Specific Antioxidants with Anti-inflammatory Properties:** Certain antioxidants have been found to possess specific anti-inflammatory properties. For instance, curcumin, a compound found in turmeric, exhibits potent anti-inflammatory effects by targeting multiple inflammation pathways.

Incorporating antioxidant-rich foods into your diet can provide you with a wide array of these beneficial compounds, which in turn can help reduce inflammation in the body. However, it's important to note that while antioxidants play a significant role in maintaining health, they are not a panacea for all ailments. A balanced lifestyle, including regular physical activity, adequate sleep, and stress management, is also essential for overall well-being

Vitamins And Minerals

Vitamins and minerals are essential nutrients that our bodies require in small amounts for proper functioning. They play crucial roles in various bodily processes, including metabolism, growth, and maintenance of overall health. While both vitamins and minerals are necessary for our well-being, they differ in their chemical structures and functions.

Vitamins are organic compounds that are required in small quantities to support normal physiological functions. They are classified into two categories: water-soluble and fat-soluble vitamins. Water-soluble vitamins, such as vitamin C and the B-complex vitamins, are not stored in the body and need to be replenished regularly through the diet. On the other hand, fat-soluble vitamins, including vitamins A, D, E, and K, can be stored in the body's fatty tissues and liver for future use.

Minerals, on the other hand, are inorganic substances that are essential for various bodily functions. They are classified into two categories: major minerals and trace minerals. Major minerals, such as calcium, phosphorus, magnesium, sodium, and potassium, are required in relatively larger amounts, whereas trace minerals, including iron, zinc, copper, selenium, and iodine, are needed in smaller quantities.

Having a well-balanced diet that includes a variety of fruits, vegetables, whole grains, lean proteins, and dairy products is crucial for obtaining an adequate intake of vitamins and minerals. However, certain individuals may have specific nutrient requirements or conditions that necessitate additional attention to certain vitamins and minerals.

Vitamin D

Vitamin D, also known as the "sunshine vitamin," is a fat-soluble vitamin that plays a vital role in maintaining overall health. It is unique compared to other vitamins because our bodies can produce it when the skin is exposed to sunlight. However, vitamin D deficiency is prevalent worldwide, and many individuals do not obtain enough through sunlight alone.

Importance Of Vitamin D For Pmr

Vitamin D is particularly important for individuals with polymyalgia rheumatica (PMR), a condition characterized by muscle pain and stiffness, especially in the shoulders, neck, and hips. Research suggests that vitamin D may have anti-inflammatory effects and can help reduce pain and inflammation associated with PMR. Furthermore, adequate vitamin D levels have been associated with improved muscle strength and function, which can be beneficial for individuals with PMR.

Sources Of Vitamin D

In addition to sunlight exposure, vitamin D can be obtained through certain dietary sources. These include:

1. **Fatty Fish**: Fatty fish such as salmon, mackerel, and trout are excellent sources of vitamin D. Consuming these fish a few times a week can contribute significantly to vitamin D intake.

2. **Egg Yolks**: Egg yolks also contain vitamin D. Including eggs in your diet can provide a small amount of this essential nutrient.

3. **Fortified Foods**: Some food products, such as milk, cereal, and orange juice, are often fortified with vitamin D. Check the labels to identify fortified options.

4. **Supplements**: If it's challenging to obtain adequate vitamin D through sunlight and diet alone, supplements can be used under the guidance of a healthcare professional.

It's important to note that while food sources can contribute to vitamin D intake, they may not provide sufficient amounts to meet the recommended daily intake, especially for individuals with specific health conditions or limited sun exposure. Regular sunlight exposure, particularly during the midday hours, allows the body to synthesize vitamin D naturally.

Optimal Vitamin D Levels

The optimal levels of vitamin D in the body are measured through a blood test that determines the concentration of 25-hydroxyvitamin D [25(OH)D]. The measurement is typically reported in nanograms per milliliter (ng/mL) or nanomoles per liter (nmol/L). The recommended optimal levels of vitamin D can vary depending on different sources and guidelines. However, generally, a level of 20-50 ng/mL (or 50-125 nmol/L) is considered adequate for most individuals.

Maintaining optimal vitamin D levels is essential for overall health and well-being. Vitamin D deficiency can lead to various health problems, including weakened bones, increased risk of fractures, muscle weakness, and impaired immune function. In addition to its role in bone health, vitamin D is involved in modulating the immune system, promoting cardiovascular health, and supporting brain function.

Several factors can affect an individual's vitamin D status. These include geographical location, time of year, skin pigmentation, age, and lifestyle factors. Individuals living in northern latitudes, where sunlight exposure is limited, may be at a higher risk of vitamin D deficiency. Similarly, people with darker skin pigmentation may have reduced vitamin D synthesis in response to sunlight.

To optimize vitamin D levels, it is recommended to follow a balanced approach that includes sunlight exposure, dietary sources, and, if necessary, supplementation. Spending around 10-30 minutes in the sun during midday, with arms and legs exposed, can help the body produce vitamin D. However, it's essential to balance sun exposure to avoid harmful effects from excessive UV radiation. People with limited sun exposure or higher risk of deficiency may benefit from vitamin D supplements.

When considering supplementation, it is advisable to consult with a healthcare professional to determine the appropriate dosage based on individual needs and health conditions. They can perform a blood test to assess vitamin D levels and provide guidance on supplementation if necessary.

Calcium

Calcium is an essential mineral that plays a crucial role in maintaining overall health and well-being. It is the most abundant mineral in the human body and is primarily stored in the bones and teeth. Apart from its structural role, calcium is involved in numerous physiological processes, such as muscle contraction, nerve transmission, blood clotting, and hormone secretion. This paragraph will delve deeper into the significance of calcium and its impact on various aspects of health.

Calcium In Pmr Management

Calcium also plays a significant role in the management of certain health conditions, including polymyalgia rheumatica (PMR). PMR is an inflammatory disorder that affects the muscles and can cause stiffness, pain, and limited range of motion, especially in the shoulders, neck, and hips. Calcium is believed to contribute to the management of PMR through its interaction with corticosteroid therapy.

Corticosteroids are commonly prescribed medications for PMR, as they help reduce inflammation and alleviate symptoms. However, long-term corticosteroid use can lead to a loss of bone density, increasing the risk of osteoporosis and fractures. Calcium supplementation, along with vitamin D, is often recommended to counteract the negative effects of corticosteroids on bone health.

By ensuring an adequate intake of calcium, individuals with PMR can support bone strength and minimize the potential bone loss associated with corticosteroid treatment. It is essential to consult with a healthcare professional to determine the appropriate dosage and form of calcium supplementation, as well as to monitor bone health regularly.

Calcium-Rich Food Sources

While calcium supplements can be beneficial in certain situations, obtaining calcium from natural food sources is generally preferred, as it offers additional nutritional benefits. There are several calcium-rich food sources that can be incorporated into a balanced diet to ensure an adequate intake of this vital mineral. Below are some examples of foods that are excellent sources of calcium:

1. **Dairy Products**: Milk, yogurt, and cheese are well-known for their high calcium content. They are also excellent sources of protein, vitamins, and minerals.

2. **Leafy Green Vegetables**: Vegetables such as spinach, kale, collard greens, and broccoli are

not only rich in calcium but also provide other essential nutrients like fiber, vitamins A, C, and K, and folate.

3. **Fish with Edible Bones**: Certain types of fish, such as canned salmon and sardines, contain edible bones that are an excellent source of calcium. These fish varieties also provide omega-3 fatty acids, which have numerous health benefits.

4. **Fortified Foods**: Some foods, such as orange juice, cereals, and plant-based milk alternatives, are often fortified with calcium. They can be good options for individuals who avoid dairy or have specific dietary restrictions.

5. **Legumes and Nuts**: Foods like almonds, chia seeds, tofu, and soybeans are not only rich in calcium but also offer plant-based protein, fiber, and other essential nutrients.

It is important to note that the bioavailability of calcium can vary across different food sources. Additionally, certain factors, such as vitamin D levels and the presence of other nutrients in the diet, can influence the absorption of calcium. Therefore, it is advisable to maintain a diverse and balanced diet that incorporates a variety of calcium-rich foods to ensure optimal calcium intake

Magnesium

Magnesium is an essential mineral that plays a crucial role in numerous physiological processes within the human body. It is involved in over 300 enzymatic reactions, contributing to the proper functioning of various systems, including nerve and muscle function, energy metabolism, protein synthesis, and DNA synthesis. This versatile mineral is vital for maintaining overall health and well-being. Let's explore the benefits of magnesium for PMR (Polymyalgia Rheumatica) and the food sources that provide this essential mineral.

Benefits Of Magnesium For Pmr

PMR is a chronic inflammatory disorder characterized by severe muscle stiffness and pain, particularly in the shoulders, neck, and hips. Magnesium has been recognized for its potential benefits in managing PMR symptoms and promoting overall joint and muscle health. Here are some ways in which magnesium can be beneficial for individuals with PMR:

1. **Muscle Relaxation:** Magnesium acts as a natural muscle relaxant, helping to alleviate muscle stiffness and reduce pain associated with PMR. It works by blocking the release of certain neurotransmitters that cause muscle

contractions, promoting a more relaxed state.

2. **Inflammation Reduction:** Magnesium possesses anti-inflammatory properties that can help mitigate the inflammatory response seen in PMR. By modulating the release of inflammatory mediators and suppressing the activity of pro-inflammatory molecules, magnesium may aid in reducing inflammation and alleviating symptoms.

3. **Pain Management:** The analgesic properties of magnesium make it valuable in managing pain related to PMR. It can help to reduce the perception of pain by blocking pain signals from reaching the brain and enhancing the release of endorphins, which are natural pain-relieving compounds.

4. **Bone Health:** Adequate magnesium levels are essential for maintaining healthy bones and preventing osteoporosis. PMR patients are often prescribed corticosteroids, which can lead to bone loss. Magnesium supplementation may help counteract the negative effects of corticosteroids and support bone density.

5. **Stress and Sleep Support:** PMR can cause sleep disturbances and increased stress levels. Magnesium plays a role in regulating the body's stress response and promoting relaxation. By aiding in the production of neurotransmitters like serotonin, magnesium may contribute to improved sleep quality and reduced stress.

Food Sources Of Magnesium

While magnesium supplements are available, it's always beneficial to obtain nutrients from natural food sources whenever possible. Here are some excellent dietary sources of magnesium:

1. **Dark Leafy Greens:** Spinach, kale, Swiss chard, and other dark leafy greens are rich in magnesium. Incorporating these greens into your diet through salads, smoothies, or cooked dishes can boost your magnesium intake.

2. **Nuts and Seeds:** Almonds, cashews, peanuts, pumpkin seeds, and sesame seeds are all excellent sources of magnesium. Snacking on a handful of nuts or incorporating them into your meals and desserts can provide a magnesium-rich boost.

3. **Whole Grains:** Whole grains like quinoa, brown rice, oats, and whole wheat contain significant amounts of magnesium. Choosing whole grain products over refined grains can enhance your magnesium intake.

4. **Legumes:** Beans, lentils, and chickpeas are not only high in fiber and protein but also provide a good amount of magnesium. Incorporate legumes into soups, stews, salads, or make them into delicious spreads like hummus.

5. **Fish and Seafood:** Some fish and seafood options are rich in magnesium. Salmon, mackerel, halibut, and tuna can be excellent choices to

increase your magnesium intake while benefiting from their omega-3 fatty acids.

6. **Bananas:** This popular fruit not only provides potassium but is also a decent source of magnesium. Enjoy bananas as a quick and nutritious snack or use them in smoothies, oatmeal, or baked goods.

7. **Avocado:** Apart from being a creamy and delicious addition to various dishes, avocados offer a good amount of magnesium. Spread avocado on toast, add it to salads or use it as a base for dips like guacamole.

8. **Dark Chocolate:** Good news for chocolate lovers! Dark chocolate with a high cocoa content is a surprising source of magnesium. Enjoy a small piece of dark chocolate as a treat while also benefiting from its antioxidants.

9. **Yogurt:** Yogurt is not only a probiotic-rich food but also contains magnesium. Choose plain, unsweetened yogurt and add your favorite fruits or a drizzle of honey for a nutritious and magnesium-rich snack.

10. **Tofu:** For those following a plant-based or vegetarian diet, tofu can be an excellent source of magnesium. Incorporate tofu into stir-fries, salads, or even use it as a substitute for meat in various recipes.

11. **Dried Fruits:** Dried fruits like figs, apricots, and raisins are concentrated sources of nutrients, including magnesium. They make for a convenient and portable snack, or you can use

them as a topping for cereals, yogurt, or salads.

It's important to note that the magnesium content in foods can vary based on factors such as soil quality and processing methods. However, incorporating a diverse range of magnesium-rich foods into your diet can help ensure an adequate intake of this essential mineral.

CHAPTER THREE

Creating an Anti-Inflammatory
Diet Plan for PMR

General Dietary Recommendations

Maintaining a healthy diet is essential for overall well-being and to support optimal bodily functions. General dietary recommendations serve as a guideline for individuals to make informed choices about their eating habits. While specific nutritional needs may vary depending on factors such as age, gender, and activity level, there are several fundamental principles that can guide everyone towards a balanced and nutritious diet.

1. **Balanced Macronutrients**: A well-rounded diet should include a balance of macronutrients, which are carbohydrates, proteins, and fats. Carbohydrates provide energy, proteins support growth and repair, and fats are important for hormone production and insulation. Aiming to consume a mix of these macronutrients helps ensure a diverse range of nutrients.

2. **Adequate Micronutrients**: In addition to macronutrients, it is crucial to obtain an adequate intake of micronutrients, such as vitamins and minerals. These nutrients are necessary for various physiological functions, including maintaining a strong immune system, promoting healthy bones, and supporting cognitive function. Consuming a variety of fruits, vegetables, whole grains, legumes, and lean proteins can help meet micronutrient needs.

3. **Portion Control**: Portion control plays a vital role in maintaining a healthy weight and preventing overeating. It involves being mindful of the quantity of food consumed and recognizing when to stop eating. Balancing portion sizes with individual energy requirements can help avoid excessive calorie intake and support weight management.

4. **Moderation**: Moderation is key when it comes to foods and beverages that are high in sugar, salt, and unhealthy fats. While it is not necessary to completely eliminate these items from the diet, consuming them in moderation can help prevent negative health effects associated with excessive intake. This approach allows for occasional treats while focusing on nutrient-dense options as the foundation of one's diet.

5. **Fiber-rich Foods**: Including fiber-rich foods, such as whole grains, fruits, vegetables, and legumes, is important for digestive health. Fiber adds bulk to the diet, aids in regular bowel movements, and promotes a feeling of fullness, which can

assist with weight management. It also helps regulate blood sugar levels and lowers the risk of certain diseases, such as heart disease and type 2 diabetes.

6. **Variety and Diversity**: Consuming a wide range of foods is crucial to ensure an adequate intake of essential nutrients. Different foods contain unique combinations of vitamins, minerals, and phytochemicals, which have diverse health benefits. Aim to incorporate a variety of colors, textures, and flavors into meals and snacks to maximize nutrient intake and enhance culinary enjoyment.

7. **Mindful Eating**: Practicing mindful eating involves paying attention to physical hunger and satiety cues, as well as the sensory aspects of food. It encourages savoring each bite, eating slowly, and being fully present during mealtimes. This approach promotes a healthier relationship with food, helps prevent overeating, and allows for a deeper appreciation of the eating experience.

8. **Individualized Approach**: While general dietary recommendations provide a framework for healthy eating, it is important to acknowledge individual differences and preferences. Factors such as cultural background, food allergies, and personal taste play a role in shaping dietary choices. Working with a registered dietitian or nutritionist can help tailor a dietary plan to meet specific needs and goals.

7 Days Sample Meal Plan

A well-planned meal plan can be an effective tool for maintaining a balanced and healthy diet. It can help you stay on track with your nutrition goals, ensure you're getting all the necessary nutrients, and make meal preparation easier. In this article, we will provide a 7-day sample meal plan that covers various meals throughout the day, offering a diverse range of flavors and nutritional benefits.

Day 1: Monday

Breakfast: Start your week with a nutritious and energizing meal. Try a bowl of oatmeal topped with sliced bananas, a sprinkle of cinnamon, and a drizzle of honey. Pair it with a cup of Greek yogurt for added protein.

Lunch: For a satisfying midday meal, prepare a colorful salad with mixed greens, cherry tomatoes, cucumber slices, grilled chicken breast, and a light vinaigrette dressing.

Afternoon Snack: Keep your energy levels up with a handful of almonds and a piece of fruit, such as an apple or orange.

Dinner: Enjoy a flavorful dinner by grilling a salmon fillet and serving it with quinoa and roasted vegetables like broccoli, bell peppers, and carrots.

Evening Snack: As a light evening snack, have a small bowl of Greek yogurt topped with a few berries and a sprinkle of granola.

Day 2: Tuesday

Breakfast: Kickstart your day with a protein-packed breakfast. Prepare scrambled eggs with spinach, mushrooms, and feta cheese. Serve it with a slice of whole-grain toast.

Lunch: Opt for a vegetarian lunch by making a chickpea and vegetable stir-fry. Sauté chickpeas, bell peppers, zucchini, and onions in olive oil and season with your favorite spices.

Afternoon Snack: Enjoy a handful of baby carrots with hummus for a crunchy and satisfying snack.

Dinner: Prepare a delicious turkey chili by combining ground turkey, kidney beans, diced tomatoes, and spices. Serve it with brown rice or a side salad.

Evening Snack: Have a cup of herbal tea and a small handful of unsalted nuts, such as almonds or walnuts.

Day 3: Wednesday

Breakfast: Start your day with a nutrient-rich smoothie. Blend together spinach, kale, a ripe banana, almond milk, and a scoop of protein powder for an extra boost.

Lunch: Prepare a wrap using whole-grain tortillas filled with grilled chicken, avocado slices, lettuce, and a drizzle of low-fat ranch dressing.

Afternoon Snack: Enjoy a handful of edamame for a protein-packed and satisfying snack.

Dinner: Make a delicious and colorful stir-fried shrimp and vegetable dish. Sauté shrimp with a mix of colorful vegetables such as bell peppers, broccoli, and snap peas. Season with soy sauce and serve over brown rice.

Evening Snack: Treat yourself to a small square of dark chocolate and a cup of herbal tea.

Day 4: Thursday

Breakfast: Whip up a batch of overnight oats by combining rolled oats, chia seeds, almond milk, and your choice of toppings such as berries, nuts, or honey. Leave it in the fridge overnight and enjoy it in the morning.

Lunch: Enjoy a light and refreshing salad by combining arugula, watermelon cubes, crumbled feta cheese, and a drizzle of balsamic glaze.

Afternoon Snack: Slice up a ripe pear and enjoy it with a spread of almond butter.

Dinner: Prepare a tasty and nutritious chicken stir-fry with a variety of colorful vegetables like snow peas, carrots, and bell peppers. Season with ginger, garlic, and low sodium soy sauce for added flavor. Serve it over a bed of brown rice or cauliflower rice.

Evening Snack: Have a handful of roasted chickpeas for a crunchy and protein-packed snack.

Day 5: Friday

Breakfast: Treat yourself to a delicious and hearty breakfast by making whole-grain pancakes topped with fresh berries and a drizzle of pure maple syrup.

Lunch: Prepare a Mediterranean-inspired salad with a base of mixed greens, cherry tomatoes, cucumber slices, Kalamata olives, feta cheese, and a lemon-herb dressing.

Afternoon Snack: Enjoy a creamy and nutritious snack by spreading some avocado on whole-grain crackers.

Dinner: Make a flavorful and colorful veggie stir-fry by sautéing tofu, broccoli florets, snap peas, and sliced bell peppers in sesame oil and soy sauce. Serve it over brown rice or noodles.

Evening Snack: Savor a small bowl of low-fat cottage cheese with a drizzle of honey and a sprinkle of cinnamon.

Day 6: Saturday

Breakfast: Start your weekend with a protein-packed

breakfast burrito. Fill a whole-grain tortilla with scrambled eggs, black beans, diced tomatoes, avocado slices, and a sprinkle of shredded cheese.

Lunch: Prepare a refreshing and filling quinoa salad by combining cooked quinoa, diced cucumbers, cherry tomatoes, feta cheese, fresh herbs, and a lemon vinaigrette.

Afternoon Snack: Enjoy a handful of trail mix made with a mix of nuts, dried fruits, and dark chocolate chips.

Dinner: Grill some lean beef or Portobello mushroom caps and serve them on whole-grain buns with lettuce, tomato slices, and a dollop of your favorite sauce.

Evening Snack: Have a bowl of sliced melon or a fruit salad for a light and hydrating evening treat.

Day 7: Sunday

Breakfast: Indulge in a leisurely breakfast by making avocado toast on whole-grain bread. Top it with sliced tomatoes, a poached egg, and a sprinkle of salt and pepper.

Lunch: Prepare a hearty and comforting lentil soup by combining cooked lentils, diced vegetables, vegetable broth, and your choice of herbs and spices.

Afternoon Snack: Enjoy a small bowl of Greek yogurt topped with fresh fruit and a drizzle of honey.

Dinner: Treat yourself to a homemade vegetable pizza using a whole-wheat crust, tomato sauce, a variety of colorful veggies like bell peppers, mushrooms, and spinach, and a sprinkle of mozzarella cheese.

Evening Snack: Enjoy a small handful of popcorn, air-popped and lightly seasoned with your favorite herbs or spices.

By following this 7-day sample meal plan, you can enjoy a variety of delicious and nutritious meals throughout the week. Remember to adjust the portion sizes and ingredients based on your personal dietary needs and preferences. It's always a good idea to consult with a healthcare professional or registered dietitian for personalized meal planning advice.

Recipes For Polymyalgia Rheumatica Diet

Grilled Salmon with Steamed Vegetables

Description: This dish combines succulent grilled salmon with a side of vibrant steamed vegetables. The salmon is seasoned with aromatic herbs and spices, resulting in a flavorful and nutritious meal.

Ingredients:

- 4 salmon fillets
- 2 tablespoons olive oil
- 1 teaspoon lemon zest
- 1 teaspoon dried dill
- Salt and pepper, to taste
- 1 cup broccoli florets
- 1 cup cauliflower florets
- 1 cup carrot slices
- 1 cup snap peas

Instructions:

1. Preheat the grill to medium-high heat.
2. In a small bowl, combine the olive oil, lemon zest, dried dill, salt, and pepper. Mix well.
3. Brush the salmon fillets with the seasoned oil mixture.
4. Grill the salmon fillets for about 4-6 minutes per side or until cooked through.
5. While the salmon is grilling, prepare the steamed vegetables.
6. Place a steamer basket in a pot filled with a small amount of water. Bring the water to a boil.
7. Add the broccoli, cauliflower, carrots, and snap peas to the steamer basket.
8. Cover the pot and steam the vegetables for 5-7 minutes or until they are tender yet still crisp.
9. Remove the steamed vegetables from the pot and serve alongside the grilled salmon.

Nutritional Information:

- Calories: 350
- Protein: 30g
- Fat: 20g
- Carbohydrates: 15g
- Fiber: 6g

Quinoa Salad with Roasted Chicken

Description: This refreshing quinoa salad features tender roasted chicken, vibrant vegetables, and a zesty dressing. It's a satisfying and nutritious meal that can be enjoyed for lunch or dinner.

Ingredients:

- 2 cups cooked quinoa
- 2 cups roasted chicken breast, shredded
- 1 cup cherry tomatoes, halved
- 1 cucumber, diced
- 1 bell pepper, diced
- 1/4 cup red onion, finely chopped
- 1/4 cup fresh parsley, chopped
- 1/4 cup fresh mint, chopped

Dressing:

- 2 tablespoons olive oil
- 1 tablespoon lemon juice
- 1 tablespoon Dijon mustard
- 1 clove garlic, minced

- Salt and pepper, to taste

Instructions:

1. In a large bowl, combine the cooked quinoa, roasted chicken breast, cherry tomatoes, cucumber, bell pepper, red onion, parsley, and mint.

2. In a separate small bowl, whisk together the olive oil, lemon juice, Dijon mustard, minced garlic, salt, and pepper to make the dressing.

3. Pour the dressing over the quinoa salad and toss gently to combine.

4. Taste and adjust the seasoning if needed.

5. Serve the quinoa salad immediately or refrigerate for later use.

Nutritional Information:

- Calories: 400
- Protein: 30g
- Fat: 15g
- Carbohydrates: 35g
- Fiber: 6g

Turkey Stir-Fry

Description: This flavorful turkey stir-fry is packed with colorful vegetables and tossed in a savory sauce. It's a quick and healthy meal that can be enjoyed any day of the week.

Ingredients:

- 1 pound turkey breast, thinly sliced

- 2 tablespoons soy sauce
- 1 tablespoon oyster sauce
- 1 tablespoon cornstarch
- 1 tablespoon vegetable oil
- 2 cloves garlic, minced
- 1 tablespoon ginger, minced
- 1 bell pepper, sliced
- 1 cup snow peas
- 1 cup broccoli florets
- 1 carrot, sliced
- 1/2 cup sliced mushrooms
- 2 green onions, chopped
- Sesame seeds, for garnish

Instructions:

1. In a small bowl, whisk together the soy sauce, oyster sauce, and cornstarch. Set aside.

2. Heat the vegetable oil in a large skillet or wok over medium-high heat.

3. Add the minced garlic and ginger to the hot oil and stir-fry for 1 minute until fragrant.

4. Add the sliced turkey breast to the skillet and cook until browned and cooked through.

5. Remove the cooked turkey from the skillet and set aside.

6. In the same skillet, add the bell pepper, snow peas, broccoli florets, carrot slices, and sliced mushrooms. Stir-fry for 3-4 minutes until the vegetables are crisp-tender.

7. Return the cooked turkey to the skillet and pour the sauce mixture over the ingredients.

8. Stir-fry for an additional 2-3 minutes until the sauce has thickened and coats the turkey and vegetables.

9. Sprinkle with chopped green onions and sesame seeds for garnish.

10. Serve the turkey stir-fry over steamed rice or noodles.

Nutritional Information:

- Calories: 300
- Protein: 25g
- Fat: 10g
- Carbohydrates: 25g
- Fiber: 6g

Baked Cod with Herbed Quinoa

Description: This baked cod dish is served with a flavorful and aromatic herbed quinoa. The tender cod fillets are seasoned and baked to perfection, complemented by the light and fluffy quinoa.

Ingredients:

- 4 cod fillets
- 2 tablespoons olive oil
- 1 teaspoon dried thyme
- 1 teaspoon dried rosemary
- Salt and pepper, to taste

- 1 cup quinoa
- 2 cups vegetable broth
- 1 tablespoon fresh parsley, chopped
- 1 tablespoon fresh lemon juice

Instructions:

1. Preheat the oven to 400°F (200°C).
2. Place the cod fillets on a baking sheet lined with parchment paper.
3. Drizzle the cod fillets with olive oil and season with dried thyme, dried rosemary, salt, and pepper.
4. Bake the cod fillets in the preheated oven for 12-15 minutes or until the fish is cooked through and flakes easily with a fork.
5. While the cod is baking, prepare the herbed quinoa.
6. Rinse the quinoa under cold water.
7. In a saucepan, bring the vegetable broth to a boil.
8. Add the rinsed quinoa to the boiling broth, reduce the heat to low, cover, and simmer for 15 minutes or until the quinoa is tender and the liquid is absorbed.
9. Fluff the cooked quinoa with a fork and stir in the fresh parsley and lemon juice.
10. Serve the baked cod fillets over a bed of herbed quinoa.

Nutritional Information:

- Calories: 250

- Protein: 25g
- Fat: 8g
- Carbohydrates: 20g
- Fiber: 3g

Lentil Soup

Description: This hearty and comforting lentil soup is packed with nutritious ingredients and warming spices. It's a satisfying meal on its own or can be served with crusty bread for a complete and wholesome dinner.

Ingredients:

- 1 cup dried lentils
- 1 tablespoon olive oil
- 1 onion, chopped
- 2 carrots, diced
- 2 celery stalks, diced
- 3 cloves garlic, minced
- 1 teaspoon ground cumin
- 1 teaspoon ground coriander
- 1/2 teaspoon turmeric
- 6 cups vegetable broth
- 1 bay leaf
- Salt and pepper, to taste
- Fresh parsley, chopped (for garnish)

Instructions:

1. Rinse the lentils under cold water and set aside.
2. In a large pot, heat the olive oil over medium heat.

3. Add the chopped onion, diced carrots, and diced celery to the pot. Sauté for 5 minutes until the vegetables start to soften.

4. Add the minced garlic, ground cumin, ground coriander, and turmeric to the pot. Stir and cook for 1 minute until fragrant.

5. Pour in the vegetable broth and add the rinsed lentils and bay leaf.

6. Bring the soup to a boil, then reduce the heat to low and simmer for about 30-40 minutes until the lentils are tender.

7. Season with salt and pepper to taste.

8. Remove the bay leaf from the soup.

9. Ladle the lentil soup into bowls and garnish with fresh chopped parsley.

10. Serve hot and enjoy the comforting flavors.

Nutritional Information:

- Calories: 200
- Protein: 10g
- Fat: 4g
- Carbohydrates: 30g
- Fiber: 10g

Grilled Chicken Breast with Sweet Potato Mash

Description: This dish features tender and juicy grilled chicken breast served with creamy sweet potato mash. The combination of flavors and textures makes it a satisfying and well-balanced meal.

Ingredients:

- 4 chicken breasts
- 2 tablespoons olive oil
- 1 teaspoon dried thyme
- 1 teaspoon paprika
- Salt and pepper, to taste
- 2 large sweet potatoes, peeled and diced
- 2 tablespoons butter
- 1/4 cup milk (or almond milk for a dairy-free option)
- Salt and pepper, to taste
- Fresh chives, chopped (for garnish)

Instructions:

1. Preheat the grill to medium-high heat.
2. In a small bowl, combine the olive oil, dried thyme, paprika, salt, and pepper. Mix well.
3. Brush the chicken breasts with the seasoned oil mixture.
4. Grill the chicken breasts for about 6-8 minutes per side or until cooked through and the internal temperature reaches 165°F (74°C).
5. While the chicken is grilling, prepare the sweet potato mash.
6. Place the diced sweet potatoes in a pot and cover with water. Bring to a boil and cook for 15-20 minutes until the sweet potatoes are tender.
7. Drain the cooked sweet potatoes and return them

to the pot.

8. Add the butter, milk, salt, and pepper to the pot.

9. Mash the sweet potatoes with a potato masher or fork until smooth and creamy.

10. Taste and adjust the seasoning if needed.

11. Serve the grilled chicken breast alongside a generous portion of sweet potato mash.

12. Garnish with fresh chopped chives for added flavor.

Nutritional Information:

- Calories: 350
- Protein: 40g
- Fat: 10g
- Carbohydrates: 25g
- Fiber: 4g

Vegetable Curry with Brown Rice

Description: This vegetable curry is a flavorful and wholesome dish that is loaded with a variety of colorful vegetables and aromatic spices. It's served with nutty brown rice for a complete and satisfying meal.

Ingredients:

- 1 tablespoon vegetable oil
- 1 onion, diced
- 2 cloves garlic, minced

- 1 tablespoon ginger, grated
- 1 tablespoon curry powder
- 1 teaspoon ground cumin
- 1 teaspoon ground coriander
- 1/2 teaspoon turmeric
- 1/2 teaspoon paprika
- 1 cup cauliflower florets
- 1 cup broccoli florets
- 1 carrot, sliced
- 1 bell pepper, diced
- 1 zucchini, diced
- 1 cup canned chickpeas, drained and rinsed
- 1 cup coconut milk
- 1 cup vegetable broth
- Salt and pepper, to taste
- Fresh cilantro, chopped (for garnish)
- Cooked brown rice, for serving

Instructions:

1. Heat the vegetable oil in a large pot or skillet over medium heat.

2. Add the diced onion, minced garlic, and grated ginger to the pot. Sauté for 2-3 minutes until the onion becomes translucent.

3. Add the curry powder, ground cumin, ground coriander, turmeric, and paprika to the pot. Stir and cook for 1 minute until the spices are fragrant.

4. Add the cauliflower florets, broccoli florets, carrot slices, diced bell pepper, diced zucchini, and

drained chickpeas to the pot. Stir to coat the vegetables with the spices.

5. Pour in the coconut milk and vegetable broth. Stir well.

6. Bring the mixture to a simmer and reduce the heat to low. Cover and cook for 15-20 minutes until the vegetables are tender.

7. Season with salt and pepper to taste.

8. Remove the pot from the heat and let it sit for a few minutes to allow the flavors to meld.

9. Serve the vegetable curry over cooked brown rice.

10. Garnish with fresh chopped cilantro for added freshness and aroma.

Nutritional Information:

- Calories: 300
- Protein: 10g
- Fat: 15g
- Carbohydrates: 40g
- Fiber: 10g

Spinach and Feta Stuffed Chicken Breast

Description: This delicious and elegant dish features tender chicken breasts stuffed with a flavorful mixture of spinach and feta cheese. It's a perfect combination of protein and greens that will impress your taste buds.

Ingredients:

- 4 chicken breasts

- 2 cups fresh spinach leaves
- 1/2 cup crumbled feta cheese
- 2 cloves garlic, minced
- 1 tablespoon olive oil
- Salt and pepper, to taste
- Toothpicks (to secure the stuffed chicken)

Instructions:

1. Preheat the oven to 375°F (190°C).

2. Slice a pocket into each chicken breast by cutting horizontally through the side of the breast, being careful not to cut all the way through.

3. In a skillet, heat the olive oil over medium heat.

4. Add the minced garlic and sauté for 1 minute until fragrant.

5. Add the fresh spinach leaves to the skillet and cook until wilted.

6. Remove the skillet from the heat and let the spinach cool slightly. 7

7. Once the spinach has cooled, squeeze out any excess liquid and transfer it to a mixing bowl.

8. Add the crumbled feta cheese to the bowl with the spinach. Season with salt and pepper to taste. Mix well to combine.

9. Spoon the spinach and feta mixture into the pockets of the chicken breasts, dividing it evenly among them.

10. Secure the openings of the chicken breasts with toothpicks to hold the stuffing in place.

11. Season the outside of the chicken breasts with salt and pepper.

12. Heat an oven-safe skillet over medium-high heat and add a drizzle of olive oil.

13. Place the stuffed chicken breasts in the skillet and sear them for about 2-3 minutes on each side until browned.

14. Transfer the skillet to the preheated oven and bake for 20-25 minutes or until the chicken is cooked through and reaches an internal temperature of 165°F (74°C).

15. Remove the skillet from the oven and let the chicken rest for a few minutes before serving.

16. Remove the toothpicks from the chicken breasts.

17. Slice the stuffed chicken breasts and serve them warm with your choice of side dishes or a fresh salad.

Nutritional Information:

- Calories: 300
- Protein: 40g
- Fat: 12g
- Carbohydrates: 2g
- Fiber: 1g

Shrimp and Vegetable Stir-Fry

Description: This vibrant stir-fry combines succulent shrimp with an array of colorful vegetables, all cooked in a delicious sauce. It's a quick and healthy meal that bursts with flavors and textures.

Ingredients:

- 1 pound shrimp, peeled and deveined
- 2 tablespoons soy sauce
- 2 tablespoons oyster sauce
- 1 tablespoon hoisin sauce
- 1 tablespoon cornstarch
- 1 tablespoon vegetable oil
- 2 cloves garlic, minced
- 1 tablespoon ginger, grated
- 1 bell pepper, sliced
- 1 cup snow peas
- 1 cup broccoli florets
- 1 carrot, sliced
- 1/2 cup sliced mushrooms
- 2 green onions, chopped
- Sesame seeds, for garnish

Instructions:

1. In a small bowl, whisk together the soy sauce, oyster sauce, hoisin sauce, and cornstarch. Set aside.

2. Heat the vegetable oil in a large skillet or wok over medium-high heat.

3. Add the minced garlic and grated ginger to the hot oil and stir-fry for 1 minute until fragrant.

4. Add the shrimp to the skillet and cook until pink and cooked through. Remove the cooked shrimp from the skillet and set aside.

5. In the same skillet, add the bell pepper, snow peas, broccoli florets, carrot slices, and sliced mushrooms. Stir-fry for 3-4 minutes until the vegetables are crisp-tender.

6. Return the cooked shrimp to the skillet and pour the sauce mixture over the ingredients.

7. Stir-fry for an additional 2-3 minutes until the sauce has thickened and coats the shrimp and vegetables.

8. Sprinkle with chopped green onions and sesame seeds for garnish.

9. Serve the shrimp and vegetable stir-fry over steamed rice or noodles.

Nutritional Information:

- Calories: 250
- Protein: 25g
- Fat: 8g
- Carbohydrates: 20g

- Fiber: 4g

Quinoa and Black Bean Salad

Description: This refreshing and nutritious salad combines protein-packed quinoa with black beans and a variety of fresh vegetables. It's a light and satisfying dish that can be enjoyed as a main course or as a side dish.

Ingredients:

- 1 cup quinoa
- 1 can black beans, drained and rinsed
- 1 red bell pepper, diced
- 1 cucumber, diced
- 1/2 red onion, finely chopped
- 1/4 cup fresh cilantro, chopped
- Juice of 1 lime
- 2 tablespoons olive oil
- 1 teaspoon cumin
- Salt and pepper, to taste
- Optional toppings: avocado slices, cherry tomatoes, feta cheese

Instructions:

1. Rinse the quinoa under cold water and cook according to package instructions. Once cooked, let it cool.

2. In a large mixing bowl, combine the cooked quinoa, black beans, diced red bell pepper, diced cucumber, finely chopped red onion, and fresh

cilantro.

3. In a small bowl, whisk together the lime juice, olive oil, cumin, salt, and pepper.

4. Pour the dressing over the quinoa mixture and toss until all the ingredients are well coated.

5. Taste and adjust the seasoning if needed.

6. Let the salad sit for at least 15 minutes to allow the flavors to meld together.

7. Before serving, you can add optional toppings such as avocado slices, halved cherry tomatoes, or crumbled feta cheese for extra flavor and texture.

8. Serve the quinoa and black bean salad chilled or at room temperature.

Nutritional Information:

- Calories: 300
- Protein: 10g
- Fat: 10g
- Carbohydrates: 40g
- Fiber: 10g

Roasted Vegetable Medley

Description: This colorful and flavorful roasted vegetable medley is a perfect side dish or can be enjoyed as a light and healthy main course. It showcases a variety of seasonal vegetables that are roasted to perfection, bringing out their natural sweetness.

Ingredients:

- 1 zucchini, sliced
- 1 yellow squash, sliced
- 1 red bell pepper, cut into strips
- 1 yellow bell pepper, cut into strips
- 1 red onion, cut into wedges
- 1 cup cherry tomatoes
- 2 tablespoons olive oil
- 2 cloves garlic, minced
- 1 teaspoon dried herbs (such as thyme, rosemary, or basil)
- Salt and pepper, to taste
- Fresh parsley, chopped (for garnish)

Instructions:

1. Preheat the oven to 425°F (220°C).

2. In a large mixing bowl, combine the sliced zucchini, sliced yellow squash, bell pepper strips, onion wedges, and cherry tomatoes.

3. Drizzle the vegetables with olive oil and sprinkle with minced garlic, dried herbs, salt, and pepper. Toss until all the vegetables are coated evenly.

4. Spread the vegetables in a single layer on a baking sheet.

5. Roast in the preheated oven for 20-25 minutes, or until the vegetables are tender and slightly caramelized, stirring halfway through.

6. Remove the roasted vegetables from the oven and transfer them to a serving dish.

7. Garnish with fresh chopped parsley for added freshness.

8. Serve the roasted vegetable medley as a side dish or as a main course with a grain or protein of your choice.

Nutritional Information:

- Calories: 150
- Protein: 4g
- Fat: 8g
- Carbohydrates: 18g
- Fiber: 6g

Grilled Tofu with Stir-Fried Bok Choy

Description: This dish features grilled tofu served with flavorful stir-fried bok choy. It's a healthy and delicious vegetarian option that provides a good balance of protein and vegetables.

Ingredients:

- 1 block of firm tofu, drained and pressed
- 2 tablespoons soy sauce
- 2 tablespoons rice vinegar
- 1 tablespoon sesame oil
- 1 tablespoon honey or maple syrup (for a vegan option)
- 2 cloves garlic, minced
- 1 tablespoon grated ginger
- 4 baby bok choy, halved
- 1 tablespoon vegetable oil
- Salt and pepper, to taste

- Toasted sesame seeds, for garnish

Instructions:

1. Preheat the grill or grill pan to medium-high heat.

2. In a shallow dish, whisk together the soy sauce, rice vinegar, sesame oil, honey or maple syrup, minced garlic, and grated ginger to make the marinade.

3. Slice the tofu into rectangular pieces and place them in the marinade. Allow the tofu to marinate for about 15 minutes, flipping once halfway through.

4. While the tofu is marinating, heat the vegetable oil in a skillet or wok over medium-high heat.

5. Add the halved baby bok choy to the skillet and stir-fry for 3-4 minutes until the bok choy is wilted but still crisp.

6. Season the bok choy with salt and pepper to taste. Remove from the heat and set aside.

7. Grill the marinated tofu for 3-4 minutes per side, or until grill marks appear and the tofu is heated through.

8. Remove the tofu from the grill and let it rest for a few minutes before slicing.

9. Slice the grilled tofu into strips.

10. Arrange the stir-fried bok choy on a serving plate and top it with the sliced grilled tofu.

11. Sprinkle with toasted sesame seeds for garnish.

12. Serve the grilled tofu with stir-fried bok choy alongside steamed rice or noodles.

Nutritional Information:

- Calories: 250
- Protein: 15g
- Fat: 12g
- Carbohydrates: 20g
- Fiber: 4g

Baked Chicken Thighs with Roasted Brussels Sprouts

Description: This hearty and flavorful dish features juicy baked chicken thighs served with roasted Brussels sprouts. It's a comforting meal that is packed with protein and nutritious vegetables.

Ingredients:

- 4 chicken thighs, bone-in and skin-on
- 1 tablespoon olive oil
- 2 teaspoons smoked paprika
- 1 teaspoon garlic powder
- 1 teaspoon dried thyme
- Salt and pepper, to taste
- 1 pound Brussels sprouts, trimmed and halved
- 2 tablespoons balsamic vinegar
- 2 tablespoons maple syrup
- 2 tablespoons melted butter or olive oil

Instructions:

1. Preheat the oven to 425°F (220°C).
2. Rub the chicken thighs with olive oil, smoked

paprika, garlic powder, dried thyme, salt, and pepper.

3. Place the chicken thighs on a baking sheet, skin side up.

4. In a separate bowl, toss the halved Brussels sprouts with balsamic vinegar, maple syrup, melted butter or olive oil, salt, and pepper.

5. Spread the Brussels sprouts around the chicken thighs on the baking sheet.

6. Bake in the preheated oven for 30-35 minutes, or until the chicken thighs are golden brown and cooked through, and the Brussels sprouts are tender and slightly caramelized.

7. Remove the baking sheet from the oven and let the chicken thighs rest for a few minutes before serving.

8. Serve the baked chicken thighs with roasted Brussels sprouts as a main course.

9. Optional: Garnish with fresh herbs such as chopped parsley or thyme for added flavor and presentation.

Nutritional Information:

- Calories: 400
- Protein: 25g
- Fat: 28g
- Carbohydrates: 15g
- Fiber: 4g

Mediterranean Salad with Grilled Shrimp

Description: This Mediterranean-inspired salad features a vibrant mix of fresh vegetables, feta cheese, olives, and grilled shrimp. It's a light and refreshing dish bursting with Mediterranean flavors.

Ingredients:

- 1 pound shrimp, peeled and deveined
- 2 tablespoons olive oil
- 1 teaspoon dried oregano
- 1 teaspoon garlic powder
- Salt and pepper, to taste
- 4 cups mixed salad greens
- 1 cup cherry tomatoes, halved
- 1 cucumber, diced
- 1/2 red onion, thinly sliced
- 1/2 cup Kalamata olives
- 1/2 cup crumbled feta cheese
- Juice of 1 lemon
- 2 tablespoons extra virgin olive oil

Instructions:

1. Preheat the grill or grill pan to medium-high heat.
2. In a bowl, combine the shrimp, olive oil, dried oregano, garlic powder, salt, and pepper. Toss to

coat the shrimp evenly.

3. Grill the shrimp for 2-3 minutes per side, or until they are pink and cooked through. Remove from the grill and set aside.

4. In a large salad bowl, combine the mixed salad greens, halved cherry tomatoes, diced cucumber, thinly sliced red onion, Kalamata olives, and crumbled feta cheese.

5. In a small bowl, whisk together the lemon juice and extra virgin olive oil to make the dressing.

6. Drizzle the dressing over the salad ingredients and toss to coat.

7. Add the grilled shrimp to the salad and gently toss to combine.

8. Serve the Mediterranean salad with grilled shrimp as a light and flavorful main course or as a side dish.

Nutritional Information:

- Calories: 300
- Protein: 25g
- Fat: 18g
- Carbohydrates: 10g
- Fiber: 3g

Vegetable Omelette

Description: This vegetable omelette is a versatile and satisfying dish that can be enjoyed for breakfast, lunch, or dinner. Packed with nutritious vegetables and protein from eggs, it's a quick and easy meal option.

Ingredients:

- 3 eggs
- 2 tablespoons milk
- Salt and pepper, to taste
- 1 tablespoon olive oil
- 1/4 cup diced onion
- 1/4 cup diced bell pepper
- 1/4 cup diced tomato
- 1/4 cup sliced mushrooms
- Handful of fresh spinach leaves
- 1/4 cup shredded cheese (such as cheddar or feta)
- Fresh herbs (such as parsley or chives) for garnish

Instructions:

1. In a bowl, whisk together the eggs, milk, salt, and pepper until well beaten.

2. Heat the olive oil in a non-stick skillet over medium heat.

3. Add the diced onion, bell pepper, tomato, and mushrooms to the skillet. Sauté for 3-4 minutes, or until the vegetables are softened.

4. Add the fresh spinach leaves to the skillet and cook for an additional minute, until wilted.

5. Pour the egg mixture over the cooked vegetables in the skillet.

6. Allow the eggs to cook undisturbed for a few minutes, until the edges start to set.

7. Gently lift the edges of the omelette with a spatula and tilt the skillet to allow the uncooked eggs to flow to the edges.

8. Sprinkle the shredded cheese evenly over one half of the omelette.

9. Carefully fold the other half of the omelette over the cheese, creating a half-moon shape.

10. Cook for another minute or until the cheese is melted and the eggs are cooked through.

11. Slide the vegetable omelette onto a plate and garnish with fresh herbs.

12. Serve the vegetable omelette hot as a standalone meal or with a side of toast or salad.

Nutritional Information:

- Calories: 250
- Protein: 15g
- Fat: 18g
- Carbohydrates: 8g
- Fiber: 2g

CHAPTER FOUR

Foods to Avoid for PMR

Inflammatory Foods

Inflammatory foods are those that can contribute to chronic inflammation in the body. Chronic inflammation has been linked to various health conditions, including heart disease, diabetes, arthritis, and certain types of cancer. By understanding which foods are inflammatory and making healthier choices, individuals can potentially reduce their risk of developing these conditions.

1. **Red and Processed Meats:** Red meats such as beef, pork, and lamb, as well as processed meats like sausages and hot dogs, have been associated with increased inflammation. These meats contain high levels of saturated fats and advanced glycation end products (AGEs), which can trigger inflammation in the body. It is advisable to limit the consumption of red and processed meats and opt for lean

protein sources like poultry, fish, and plant-based proteins.

2. Refined Grains: Refined grains, such as white bread, white rice, and pasta made from refined flour, have had their bran and germ removed, stripping them of their fiber and nutrients. These refined grains cause a rapid spike in blood sugar levels, leading to increased production of pro-inflammatory molecules in the body. Choosing whole grains like brown rice, quinoa, and whole wheat bread can help reduce inflammation due to their higher fiber and nutrient content.

3. Vegetable Oils: Certain vegetable oils, such as corn, soybean, and sunflower oils, are high in omega-6 fatty acids. While omega-6 fatty acids are essential for the body, an imbalance between omega-6 and omega-3 fatty acids can promote inflammation. Most Western diets already contain an excess of omega-6 fatty acids, so it is important to moderate the use of these oils and incorporate healthier alternatives like olive oil, avocado oil, or coconut oil.

4. Sugary Foods: Foods high in refined sugars, including desserts, sodas, and sweetened beverages, can contribute to inflammation. These sugary foods lead to spikes in blood sugar levels and trigger the release of pro-inflammatory cytokines in the body. Consuming excessive amounts of sugar has also been associated with weight gain and increased risk of chronic diseases. Reducing the intake of sugary foods and opting for natural sweeteners like honey or fruits can help mitigate inflammation.

5. Processed and Fast Foods: Processed foods such as chips, snack bars, and frozen meals often contain high levels of unhealthy fats, refined grains, and additives. These foods are typically low in nutrients and high in calories, contributing to inflammation and other health problems. Fast food items, in particular, are often fried in unhealthy oils and contain high amounts of sodium, which can further promote inflammation. Choosing whole, unprocessed foods and cooking meals at home using fresh ingredients can help reduce inflammation and improve overall health.

6. Alcohol and Sugary Drinks: Excessive alcohol consumption has been linked to inflammation in the body. Alcohol can disrupt the gut microbiota, leading to increased intestinal permeability and the release of inflammatory substances. Additionally, sugary drinks like cocktails, sweetened mixers, and even some fruit juices can contribute to inflammation due to their high sugar content. Moderation is key, and it is advisable to limit alcohol intake and opt for healthier beverage choices like water, herbal tea, or freshly squeezed juices.

Incorporating an anti-inflammatory diet, which includes a variety of fruits, vegetables, whole grains, lean proteins, and healthy fats, can help reduce chronic inflammation in the body. It is important to note that individual responses to specific foods may vary, and it can be beneficial to consult with a healthcare professional or registered dietitian for personalized dietary recommendations. By making informed food choices, individuals can support their overall health and well-being by reducing inflammation in the body.

Trans Fats And Hydrogenated Oils

Trans fats and hydrogenated oils are widely recognized as harmful components in the modern diet. These types of fats are artificially created through a process called hydrogenation, which involves adding hydrogen atoms to vegetable oils to make them more solid and increase their shelf life. However, the consumption of trans fats and hydrogenated oils has been strongly linked to various health issues, making it important to understand their impact and make healthier choices.

1. **Increased Risk of Heart Disease:** Trans fats and hydrogenated oils have been shown to raise levels of low-density lipoprotein (LDL) cholesterol, commonly known as "bad" cholesterol, while simultaneously lowering high-density lipoprotein (HDL) cholesterol, known as "good" cholesterol. This imbalance in cholesterol levels significantly increases the risk of developing heart disease, clogged arteries, and other cardiovascular problems.

2. **Inflammation and Chronic Diseases:** Trans fats and hydrogenated oils promote inflammation within the body.

They trigger the release of pro-inflammatory cytokines, contributing to chronic inflammation, which is associated with several health conditions, including heart disease, diabetes, obesity, and even certain types of cancer. Chronic inflammation can also exacerbate symptoms of autoimmune disorders, such as rheumatoid arthritis.

3. Adverse Effects on Blood Vessels: Trans fats and hydrogenated oils negatively affect blood vessel health. They can damage the inner lining of blood vessels, leading to the formation of plaques and increasing the risk of atherosclerosis. Atherosclerosis restricts blood flow and can ultimately result in heart attacks, strokes, and other cardiovascular complications.

4. Impaired Brain Function: Studies have suggested a connection between trans fats and impaired brain function. The consumption of these fats has been associated with an increased risk of cognitive decline, memory problems, and an elevated likelihood of developing neurodegenerative diseases, such as Alzheimer's disease. These detrimental effects on brain health highlight the importance of avoiding trans fats and hydrogenated oils.

5. Regulatory Efforts: Recognizing the harmful effects of trans fats, many countries and regions have implemented regulations to limit or ban their use in food products. This has led to a significant reduction in trans fat consumption in some areas. However, it is still crucial for individuals to read food labels carefully and avoid products that contain partially hydrogenated oils or trans fats.

6. Choosing Healthier Alternatives: To avoid trans fats and hydrogenated oils, it is important to be mindful of the types of fats used in food preparation. Opting for healthier fats such as olive oil, avocado oil, or coconut oil can provide essential fatty acids and beneficial compounds without the harmful effects of trans fats. Additionally, incorporating foods rich in omega-3 fatty acids, such as fatty fish, flaxseeds, and walnuts, can help balance the ratio of omega-3 to omega-6 fatty acids in the diet.

Awareness and education are key to making healthier choices and reducing the consumption of trans fats and hydrogenated oils. Reading nutrition labels, selecting whole foods over processed ones, and opting for cooking methods that minimize the use of unhealthy fats can contribute to a more heart-healthy and inflammation-reducing diet. By eliminating or minimizing trans fats and hydrogenated oils, individuals can support their overall well-being and reduce the risk of developing chronic diseases.

Refined Sugars And High-Fructose Corn Syrup

Refined sugars and high-fructose corn syrup (HFCS)

are common sweeteners found in many processed and packaged foods. While sugar is naturally present in various foods like fruits and dairy products, the excessive consumption of refined sugars and HFCS has been linked to a range of negative health effects. Understanding the impact of these sweeteners can help individuals make more informed dietary choices.

1. Increased Risk of Obesity: Refined sugars and HFCS are high in calories but low in nutrients. They provide empty calories, meaning they contribute to weight gain without offering any substantial nutritional value. Frequent consumption of sugary foods and beverages can lead to an excessive calorie intake, increasing the risk of obesity and related health conditions.

2. Elevated Blood Sugar Levels: Refined sugars and HFCS cause a rapid spike in blood sugar levels due to their high glycemic index. This can lead to insulin resistance over time, a condition in which cells become less responsive to the hormone insulin. Insulin resistance is associated with the development of type 2 diabetes and metabolic syndrome.

3. Increased Risk of Heart Disease: Diets high in refined sugars and HFCS have been linked to an increased risk of heart disease. The excessive intake of these sweeteners can contribute to elevated levels of triglycerides, LDL cholesterol, and blood pressure, all of which are risk factors for cardiovascular problems.

4. Dental Health Issues: Sugar is a primary contributor to tooth decay. When consumed in excess, refined sugars and HFCS provide a food source for harmful bacteria in the mouth, leading to the production of acids that erode tooth enamel. This can result in cavities, tooth sensitivity, and other dental health issues.

5. Addiction-like Properties: Some research suggests that refined sugars and HFCS can have addictive properties, leading to cravings and overconsumption. The brain's reward system can be activated by the pleasurable taste of sugar, creating a cycle of craving and consumption that can be difficult to break.

6. Hidden Sources in Processed Foods: Refined sugars and HFCS are often hidden in processed and packaged foods, making it challenging to avoid them entirely. Common culprits include sugary beverages, desserts, cereals, condiments, and even savory snacks. Reading food labels and being aware of alternative names for sugar (such as sucrose, glucose, fructose, dextrose, and maltose) can help identify and limit their intake.

Reducing the consumption of refined sugars and HFCS can have significant health benefits. Here are some strategies to achieve this:

- **Choose whole foods:** Opt for whole fruits instead of processed fruit juices, and select minimally processed foods without added sugars.
- **Cook and bake at home:** By preparing meals and

snacks at home, you have better control over the ingredients, allowing you to reduce or replace refined sugars with healthier alternatives like natural sweeteners, such as honey or maple syrup.

- **Read food labels:** Check the ingredient lists on packaged foods to identify added sugars or alternative names for sugar. Be aware that sugar can be present in products labeled as "low-fat" or "diet" to enhance flavor.

It's important to note that naturally occurring sugars in whole foods like fruits and dairy products are not of concern, as they come packaged with essential nutrients and fiber that help mitigate their impact on blood sugar levels. However, moderation is still advised.

By reducing the consumption of refined sugars and HFCS, individuals can support their overall health, manage weight more effectively, and reduce the risk of chronic diseases such as obesity, type 2 diabetes, and heart disease.

Potential Food Sensitivities

Food sensitivities refer to adverse reactions that occur when certain foods are consumed. These reactions are different from food allergies, which involve an immune response. Food sensitivities are more commonly associated with non-immune reactions, such as digestive issues or intolerances. In this article, we will explore three common categories of potential food sensitivities: gluten and wheat products, dairy products, and nightshade vegetables.

Gluten and Wheat Products

Gluten is a protein found in wheat, barley, and rye. Some individuals may experience sensitivities or intolerances to gluten, which can lead to a range of symptoms. The most severe form of gluten sensitivity is known as celiac disease, an autoimmune disorder. Celiac disease is characterized by the immune system's reaction to gluten, leading to inflammation and damage to the small intestine.

Here are a few key points to understand about gluten sensitivity:

1. **Celiac Disease:** People with celiac disease must strictly avoid gluten in their diet to prevent damage to their intestines. Symptoms of celiac disease include diarrhea, abdominal pain, bloating, fatigue, and weight loss.

2. **Non-Celiac Gluten Sensitivity:** Some individuals may experience symptoms similar to celiac disease without having the autoimmune response. This condition is known as non-celiac gluten sensitivity. Symptoms can include bloating, gas, diarrhea, and fatigue.

3. **Wheat Allergy:** Another condition related to wheat is a wheat allergy, which is an immune response triggered by specific proteins in wheat. Wheat allergy symptoms can range from mild to severe, including hives, itching, swelling,

difficulty breathing, and even anaphylaxis in rare cases.

For individuals with gluten sensitivity, adopting a gluten-free diet is essential. This involves avoiding wheat, barley, and rye products, including bread, pasta, cereals, and baked goods. Thankfully, there is now a wide range of gluten-free alternatives available in most grocery stores, making it easier for those with sensitivities to still enjoy a varied diet.

Dairy Products

Dairy products, such as milk, cheese, and yogurt, contain lactose, a natural sugar present in milk. Lactose intolerance is a common food sensitivity where the body has difficulty digesting lactose due to a deficiency in the enzyme lactase. This deficiency leads to digestive symptoms when consuming dairy products.

Let's delve into a few important aspects of lactose intolerance:

1. **Digestive Symptoms:** Lactose intolerance can cause symptoms like bloating, gas, diarrhea, and abdominal pain after consuming dairy products. The severity of symptoms can vary among individuals, with some experiencing mild discomfort and others facing more significant issues.

2. **Primary Lactose Intolerance:** This is the most common type of lactose intolerance and is typically inherited. It occurs when the body naturally produces less lactase as a person ages.

> People with primary lactose intolerance often find it beneficial to limit or avoid dairy products to manage their symptoms.

3. **Secondary Lactose Intolerance:** In some cases, lactose intolerance can be secondary to other conditions, such as gastrointestinal infections, celiac disease, or inflammatory bowel diseases. Treating the underlying condition can help alleviate lactose intolerance symptoms.

Fortunately, there are numerous dairy alternatives available for individuals with lactose intolerance. These include lactose-free milk, plant-based milks (such as almond, soy, or oat milk), and dairy-free yogurts and cheeses. These alternatives offer options for those who wish to avoid dairy while still enjoying similar products.

Nightshade Vegetables

Nightshade vegetables belong to the Solanaceae family and include popular foods like tomatoes, potatoes, eggplants, and peppers. While these vegetables are nutritious and widely consumed, some individuals may have sensitivity to its consumption.

Let's explore some key points regarding nightshade vegetable sensitivities:

1. **Alkaloids:** Nightshade vegetables contain alkaloids, natural compounds that may affect some individuals. One of the most well-known alkaloids found in nightshades is solanine. Sensitivity to solanine or other alkaloids can lead

to symptoms in certain individuals.

2. **Symptoms:** Sensitivities to nightshade vegetables can manifest in various ways, including digestive issues, joint pain, inflammation, skin rashes, or worsening of symptoms in conditions like arthritis or autoimmune diseases. However, it's important to note that the majority of people can consume nightshade vegetables without experiencing any adverse effects.

3. **Individual Variation:** Sensitivity to nightshade vegetables can vary greatly among individuals. What may cause symptoms in one person might not affect another person at all. It is important to listen to your body and pay attention to any adverse reactions you may have after consuming these vegetables.

If you suspect that you have a nightshade vegetable sensitivity, it can be helpful to keep a food diary to track your symptoms and identify any patterns or triggers. If you notice a consistent reaction after consuming nightshades, it may be worth consulting with a healthcare professional or registered dietitian for further evaluation and guidance.

It's important to note that eliminating entire food groups, such as nightshade vegetables, should be done under the guidance of a healthcare professional or registered dietitian, as it can potentially lead to nutrient deficiencies. They can help ensure that you maintain a balanced and nutritious diet while managing your sensitivities.

CONCLUSION

Summary of key points

Following a PMR-friendly (Plant-based Mediterranean Diet) diet can have numerous health benefits and is a sustainable approach to nourishing your body. This diet combines the principles of the Mediterranean diet, which is known for its heart-healthy properties, with a plant-based focus, emphasizing whole foods derived from plants. The key points to consider when adopting a PMR-friendly diet are:

1. **Plant-based emphasis:** The PMR-friendly diet places a strong emphasis on consuming plant-based foods, such as fruits, vegetables, whole grains, legumes, nuts, and seeds. These foods provide a rich array of nutrients, including vitamins, minerals, fiber, and antioxidants, which promote overall health and reduce the risk of chronic diseases.

2. **Incorporation of healthy fats:** The Mediterranean aspect of the PMR-friendly diet encourages the consumption of healthy fats, primarily derived from plant sources such as olive oil, avocados, and nuts. These fats are known to support heart

health, improve cholesterol levels, and provide satiety, making the diet enjoyable and satisfying.

3. **Moderate consumption of animal products:** While the PMR-friendly diet is primarily plant-based, it allows for moderate consumption of animal products, such as fish, poultry, dairy, and eggs. However, it is recommended to choose lean sources of animal protein and prioritize fish, especially fatty fish rich in omega-3 fatty acids, which have numerous health benefits.

4. **Reduced intake of processed foods:** A key principle of the PMR-friendly diet is minimizing the consumption of processed foods, which are typically high in added sugars, unhealthy fats, and sodium. Instead, the focus is on whole, unprocessed foods that are nutrient-dense and support optimal health.

5. **Enjoyment of meals and social connections:** The PMR-friendly diet not only promotes physical health but also emphasizes the enjoyment of meals and the cultivation of social connections. Sharing meals with family and friends, savoring the flavors of whole foods, and practicing mindful eating are integral aspects of this diet.

By following a PMR-friendly diet, you can experience a wide range of benefits, including improved cardiovascular health, weight management, reduced risk of chronic diseases (such as diabetes, certain cancers, and neurodegenerative disorders), increased energy levels, and overall well-being.

Encouragement And Motivation For Following A Pmr-Friendly Diet

Embarking on a new dietary approach can sometimes feel challenging, but the PMR-friendly diet offers a wealth of encouragement and motivation to help you succeed in adopting this lifestyle. Here are some key factors that can inspire and support your journey:

1. **Health benefits:** The PMR-friendly diet has been extensively studied and shown to have numerous health benefits. These include reducing the risk of heart disease, improving blood pressure and cholesterol levels, promoting weight loss and weight management, and enhancing overall longevity. Keeping these benefits in mind can serve as a powerful motivator to make positive changes in your eating habits.

2. **Diverse and delicious meals:** One of the exciting aspects of the PMR-friendly diet is the wide range of plant-based foods and flavors it incorporates. From colorful salads and hearty grain bowls to vibrant vegetable stir-fries and delicious legume-based dishes, there are endless possibilities to explore. Experimenting with new recipes and discovering the delicious flavors of whole foods can make the transition enjoyable and exciting.

3. **Sustainability and environmental impact:** Choosing a PMR-friendly diet aligns with sustainability and reduces your environmental

footprint. Plant-based diets have been shown to have lower greenhouse gas emissions, require less land and water resources, and contribute to the preservation of biodiversity. Knowing that your food choices can positively impact the planet can be a strong motivating factor.

4. **Community support and resources:** Joining communities and finding support from like-minded individuals can greatly enhance your motivation to follow a PMR-friendly diet. Look for online forums, social media groups, or local meetups where you can connect with others who share your dietary goals. These communities can provide a platform for sharing recipes, tips, and success stories, as well as offer a space for seeking guidance and encouragement during challenging times.

5. **Improved well-being:** Adopting a PMR-friendly diet can lead to an overall improvement in your well-being. Many people report increased energy levels, better digestion, improved mood, and enhanced mental clarity when following this lifestyle. These positive changes can serve as powerful motivators to continue making healthy choices and sticking to the diet long-term.

6. **Gradual transition and flexibility:** It's important to remember that transitioning to a PMR-friendly diet doesn't have to be an all-or-nothing approach. You can start by incorporating more plant-based meals into your routine and gradually reducing the consumption of animal products and processed foods. Additionally, the

PMR-friendly diet offers flexibility, allowing for occasional indulgences or modifications to accommodate personal preferences or social situations. This adaptability can make the diet more sustainable and easier to follow in the long run.

7. **Tracking progress and celebrating milestones:** Keeping track of your progress and celebrating milestones along the way can help you stay motivated. Set achievable goals, such as increasing the number of plant-based meals per week or trying new recipes, and track your progress. Celebrate your achievements, no matter how small, as each step forward contributes to your overall success.

8. **Education and learning:** Educating yourself about the benefits of a PMR-friendly diet and the science behind it can provide a solid foundation of knowledge and motivation. Read books, watch documentaries, and follow reputable online sources to deepen your understanding of the diet and its impact on health. The more informed you are, the more empowered and motivated you will feel to make informed food choices.

9. **Self-reflection and self-care:** Remember to practice self-reflection and self-care throughout your journey. Understand that change takes time, and it's important to be kind to yourself during any setbacks or challenges. Prioritize self-care activities that help reduce stress, such as meditation, exercise, or engaging in hobbies you enjoy. Taking care of your overall well-being will

support your motivation to maintain a PMR-friendly diet.

10. **Celebrate variety and creativity:** Embrace the diversity of plant-based foods and enjoy the opportunity to get creative in the kitchen. Explore new ingredients, experiment with different cooking methods, and try recipes from various cuisines. By celebrating the variety and flavors of plant-based meals, you'll find joy in the process and be more motivated to continue your PMR-friendly journey.

Additional Resources And References

If you're interested in further exploring the PMR-friendly diet and seeking additional resources, here are some references to get you started:

1. Books:
   - "The Plant-Based Mediterranean Diet: A Delicious Way to Eat Healthy" by Melissa DeMayo
   - "The Mediterranean Diet for Beginners: The Complete Guide - 40 Delicious Recipes, 7-Day Diet Meal Plan, and 10 Tips for Success" by Rockridge Press

2. Documentaries:
   - "Forks Over Knives" directed by Lee

Fulkerson

- "The Game Changers" directed by Louie Psihoyos

3. Websites and online communities:
    - Oldways Mediterranean Foods Alliance (https://oldwayspt.org/)
    - Plant-Based Mediterranean Diet Facebook Group (https://www.facebook.com/groups/PBMdiet)

4. Scientific papers and studies:
    - Sofi F, et al. (2014). Adherence to Mediterranean diet and health outcomes: a systematic review and meta-analysis. The American Journal of Clinical Nutrition, 99(6), 1344-1356.

- Martinez-Gonzalez MA, et al. (2019). A 14-item Mediterranean diet assessment tool and obesity indexes among high-risk subjects: the PREDIMED trial. PLoS ONE, 14(10), e0222383.

- Dinu M, et al. (2017). Vegetarian, vegan diets and multiple health outcomes: A systematic review with meta-analysis of observational studies. Critical Reviews in Food Science and Nutrition, 57(17), 3640-3649.

Remember to consult with a healthcare professional or registered dietitian before making any significant dietary changes to ensure it aligns with your individual health needs and considerations.

www.ingramcontent.com/pod-product-compliance
Lightning Source LLC
Chambersburg PA
CBHW060747260726
48660CB00002B/514